For Health

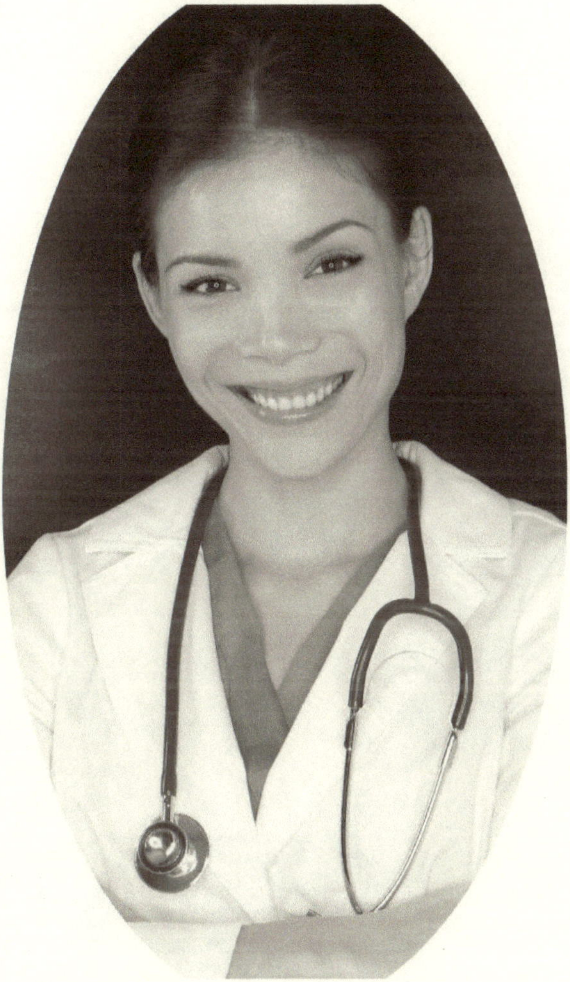

For Health

by: *Timothy Swiss*

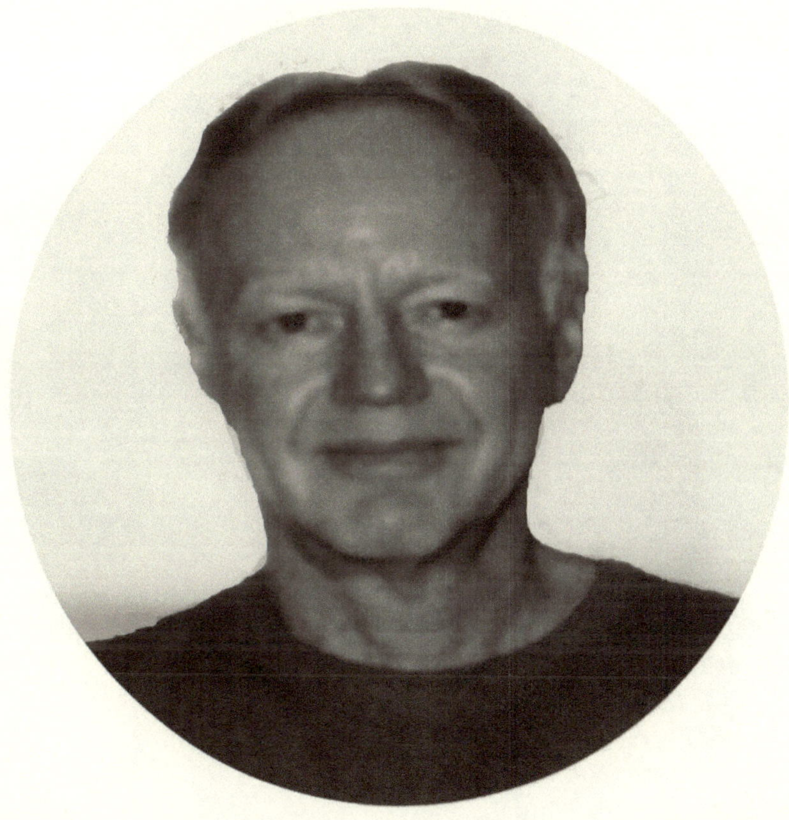

Preface

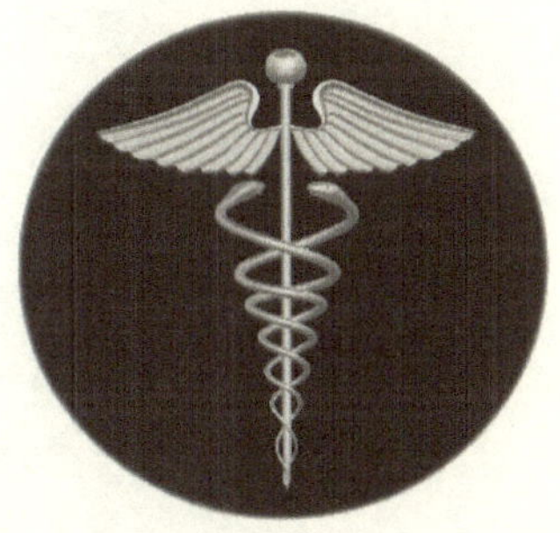

The primary purpose of this book is to provide simple instructions for clearing cyanide from one's body. The treatments for doing so are remarkably safe and inexpensive, but cyanide is not safe. Testimonials from persons who have experienced improvements from conditions such as chronic fatigue and fibromyalgia are presented, word for word, as penned by those individuals. How airborne cyanide can cause illnesses such as fibromyalgia, autism, diabetes, autoimmune diseases, myalgic encephalomyelitis, systemic exertional intolerance disease, and chronic fatigue syndrome is expounded in this book's concluding chapters. In regard to our modern, industrialized atmosphere; we all breathe cyanide, and we do so on a daily basis.

Production of hydrogen cyanide in the United States in 2003 was 2.019 billion pounds according to TOXICOLOGICAL PROFILE FOR CYANIDE, U.S. Department of Health and Human Services, Agency for Toxic Substance and Disease Registry, July, 2006. This same agency reported that the worldwide emissions of hydrogen cyanide and acetonitrile (*most of the cyanide in the atmosphere is present as hydrogen cyanide*) due to biomass burning are based in part on highly uncertain global estimates, but are estimated at about 1.1 to 3.7 billion pounds per year. This agency also reported that the half-life of hydrogen cyanide in the atmosphere is about 1 to 3 years. *Half-life of cyanide in the atmosphere* refers to the time that passes before half of a quantity of cyanide released into the atmosphere is no longer present there. Most airborne cyanide remains in the lower atmosphere, namely the air we breathe. Sensitivity to airborne cyanide varies greatly from person to person, and may sometimes be hereditary.

Table of Contents

First, sodium thiosulfate has been used for many years as an antidote for cyanide poisoning and is notably safe, with up to 12.5 grams of the injectable sodium thiosulfate having been given intravenously without ill effects [Gosselin RE, Smith RP, Hodge HC. *Clinical Toxicology of Commercial Products*, fifth edition. Baltimore/London: Williams & Wilkins; 1984, page II-125]. Next, in regard to alpha ketoglutaric acid, the author extends a special thanks to James C. Norris, Ph.D., Diplomate of the American Board of Toxicology, and Eurotox Registered Toxicologist. Alpha ketoglutaric acid is an effective antidote to cyanide poisoning and is a natural component of the Krebs cycle within the cells of the human body. Another effective antidote to cyanide poisoning is hydroxocobalamin. Hydroxocobalamin is safe to use, with a usual adult dose of five grams given intravenously over fifteen minutes for acute cyanide poisoning [note that five grams is equal to 5,000 milligrams]. Methylcobalamin, another safe form of vitamin B12, is one of the *active* forms of vitamin B12 within the body, and methylcobalamin binds cyanide [*The reaction between methylcobalamin and cyanide revisited*, Inorganica Chimica Acta, Volume 348, 15 May 2003, Pages 221-224].

<u>Chapter One</u>
Treatment for Environmental Cyanide Sensitivity

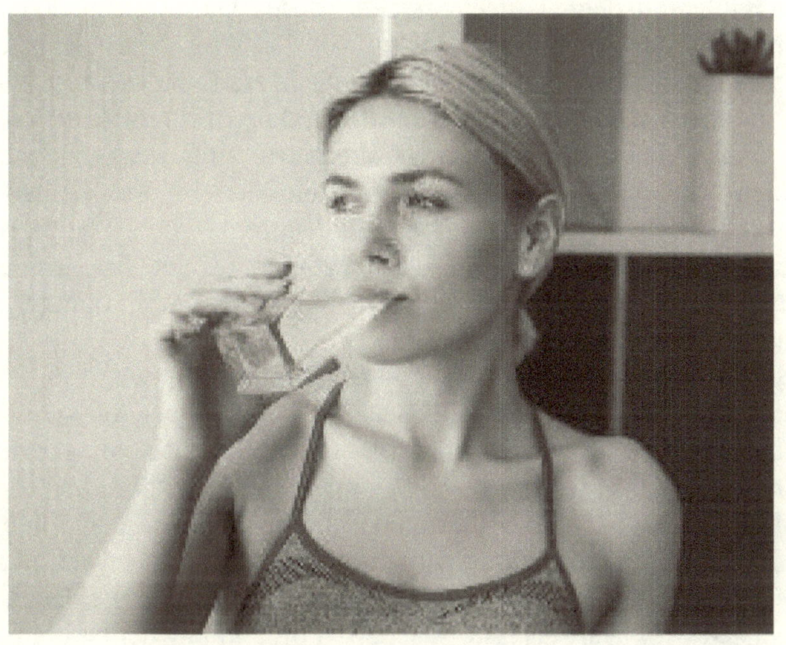

Sodium Thiosulfate Pentahydrate
(Also sold as: Sodium Thiosulfate 5H2O or Na2S2O3 5H2O)

This antidote for airborne cyanide sensitivity may be acquired at health food stores or per the internet by doing a search for Sodium Thiosulfate Pentahydrate. It is available on Amazon, and one may acquire 99.5% pure sodium thiosulfate pentahydrate very inexpensively. Larger crystals may be crushed into powder with a food processor.

<u>Dose</u>: Take 1/64th to 1/32nd tsp (*a pinch*) of sodium thiosulfate pentahydrate every two to three hours. Doses do not need to be exact. Either dissolve it in water and drink it or let it dissolve under your tongue. The half-life of sodium thiosulfate in the bloodstream may be as little as twenty minutes, and this is why doses are taken frequently. Another reason to take frequent, small doses is because a large dose would likely result in diarrhea. If this treatment causes gas or diarrhea to an intolerable degree, then try smaller doses. During sleep, do not set your alarm and awaken yourself to take doses of sodium thiosulfate pentahydrate; rather, simply start doses again after you wake up. A dose may be taken if you get up during the middle of the night to use the bathroom. Although the author is allergic to sulfa drugs, he has no problem taking this sulfur-containing antidote. In fact, he has not missed a single day taking this antidote since 1994, and he carries a sufficient quantity for several days within a Ziploc bag inside his pocket. Many people have reported feeling better within minutes after taking the first doses of this antidote.

Sulfur-containing amino acids—in combination with 50 mg of vitamin B6, 400 mcg of folic acid, and 5,000 mcg of sublingual methylcobalamin (a type of B12) or 5,000 mcg of sublingual hydroxocobalamin (a type of B12)—may be taken before bed to help the body detoxify cyanide throughout the night. Be sure and take the B6, B12, and folic acid along with the amino acids to decrease chances of elevated homocysteine levels. Elevated homocysteine levels are associated with heart disease. A scoop of protein powder before bed is one way to obtain sulfur-containing amino acids, and one may also obtain N-acetyl-cysteine capsules, taurine capsules, and L-methionine capsules. Nuts are a good food for health, and are especially good for persons with cyanide sensitivity since nuts; such as cashews, peanuts, pine nuts, pistachios, walnuts, almonds, and macadamia nuts; contain appreciable amounts of sulfur-containing amino acids. Sesame seeds are another good source of sulfur-containing amino acids. Also, since certain keto acids play a role in detoxifying cyanide, it may be beneficial to take a dose of MCT oil before bed.

In regard to sodium thiosulfate, the author has always used the sodium thiosulfate pentahydrate, never the anhydrous sodium thiosulfate. He does not advise the use of anhydrous sodium thiosulfate.

Some persons may only want to take sodium thiosulfate pentahydrate that is officially approved as a food product, even if doing so is somewhat more expensive. ACS grade is considered okay for food or drug use, and meets or surpasses standards set by the American Chemical Society (ACS). Reagent grade is also okay for food or drug use, generally being equal to ACS grade. USP grade is likewise okay for food or drug use, as is NF grade. Food grade salt is typically 99.7% to 99.99% pure, and the author has found sodium thiosulfate pentahydrate on Amazon that is a minimum of 99.5% pure, and is very inexpensive; and it is stated on this product's bottle that it is *not a hazardous substance*. The URL for this product is: https://www.amazon.com/Sodium-Thiosulfate-Crystals-99-5-Grams/dp/B00JERVY5A/ref=sr_1_3?crid=353PJYP077HRQ&keywo rds=Sodium+thiosulfate+pentahydrate&qid=1676814328&sprefix=so dium+thiosulfate+pentahydr%2Caps%2C636&sr=8-3 Or, enter *ChemCenter sodium thiosulfate pentahydrate* in the search bar on Amazon.

Of interest, a report that appeared in a neurological journal— *Medical uses of Sodium thiosulfate*, McGeer PL, McGeer EG, Lee M. J Neurol Neuromedicine (2016) 1(3): 28-30—suggests that sodium thiosulfate pentahydrate may likely decrease chances of Alzheimer's disease, and may also decrease chances of Parkinson's disease. In regard to Alzheimer's disease, the brain is the most sensitive organ in the body to hypoxia (*lack of oxygen*), and lack of oxygen can result in inflammation, and inflammation of the brain is associated with Alzheimer's disease. Cyanide causes *histotoxic hypoxia*, which is *deficient use of oxygen on the cellular level*; and therefore, cyanide appears suspicious as an underlying cause of Alzheimer's disease. And in regard to Parkinson's disease, the following internet site—

https://www.orpha.net/consor/cgi-bin/Disease_Search.php?lng=EN&data_id=21253

—contains the following statement: *Cyanide-induced parkinsonism is a rare parkinsonian syndrome due to intoxication which develops in individuals surviving an acute cyanide intoxication episode or due to chronic exposure to small cyanide doses*. It may be, perhaps, that cyanide-induced parkinsonism due to chronic exposure to small doses of cyanide is not so rare, after all.

Alpha Ketoglutaric Acid

This natural organic acid may be acquired at health food stores or through the internet. It is quite inexpensive from Trafa Rx (Canada). Just do a search for trafarx.com, and then enter alpha ketoglutaric acid in the search bar of that site. Although alpha ketoglutaric acid may be written with a hyphen, *alpha-ketoglutaric acid*, do not use the hyphen when doing a search for the product on trafarx.com. The author recommends that you acquire the alpha ketoglutaric acid rather than alpha ketoglutarate.

Alpha ketoglutaric acid is a potent antidote for treating cyanide intoxication and works synergistically (*very good combined effect*) with sodium thiosulfate pentahydrate. The alpha ketoglutaric acid and sodium thiosulfate pentahydrate may be taken at the same time, but you may want to take them separately due to the taste that results when they are mixed. The author has no problem drinking the mixture of the two.

The author recommends one-eighth teaspoon (about 563 mg) of alpha ketoglutaric acid in eight ounces of water three times daily, in the middle of each meal. Smaller doses may be used, but take at least one-sixteenth teaspoon. If your stomach tolerates the acid drink well, you may also take doses between meals, for up to six doses daily; but heartburn may occur if taking doses on an empty stomach. Take doses at least two hours apart. The author recommends swishing and swallowing a mouthful of water after each dose.

Drinking acidic drinks on a regular basis, such as sodas, may tend to dissolve calcium from teeth. This is of most concern if you sip the drink continuously throughout the day. Alpha ketoglutaric acid is an acidic drink, so swishing the mouth with water after each dose is recommended with thought for protecting the enamel on teeth.

Vital B12 Injections

Medical Provider: Date________________

Patient's Phone___________________

Patient: _________________________________   DOB: ___________

Rx: 25 mg/cc Vitamin B12 as—12.5 mg hydroxocobalamin/12.5 mg methylcobalamin.

Quantity: 10 cc (Or up to 45 cc, or a single test dose of 0.5 cc)

Sig: 0.3 cc SC (subcutaneously) or IM (intramuscularly) every 3 days (or up to 1 cc every 3 days). (Doses may also be increased up to 0.5 cc daily.)

Signature of Provider:

____

Refills: _PRN – one year_
(Note: may also have 30 to 90 [or 1] of the B12 syringes and needles if requested.)

The injectable Vital B12 requires a medical prescription and may be acquired through compounding pharmacies. This particular formula for injectable vitamin B12 has been named Vital B12 by the author. The storage life of Vital B12 has been reported as three months. It should be kept refrigerated, although it will last a couple of weeks without refrigeration. The usual dose is anywhere from 0.3 cc every three days to 0.5 cc daily. It may be injected either subcutaneously or intramuscularly. In the inconceivably harmful event that the FDA ever makes injectable methylcobalamin illegal, then the author recommends using the same amount of injectable B12, but solely as the hydroxocobalamin form of vitamin B12.

When using this product to treat illness from exposure to environmental cyanide, it is also recommended that an individual take vitamin B6, 100 mg daily in divided doses, such as 50 mg am and pm, or else 25 mg am, 25 mg at noon, and 50 mg before bed. In addition, take folic acid, 400 mcg am and pm; and vitamin D3, 1,000 IU daily. If advised by a doctor, take larger daily doses of vitamin D3. Many persons may need 3,000 IU daily or even 5,000 IU daily of vitamin D3 to maintain proper vitamin D3 levels.

Persons taking Vital B12 injections less frequently, such as once every 3 days, may supplement their B12 intake with methylcobalamin 5,000 mcg sublingual tablets and/or hydroxocobalamin 5,000 mcg sublingual tablets, taking one tablet sublingually each morning and one tablet sublingually each evening. The sublingual methylcobalamin and/or sublingual hydroxocobalamin may also be used by persons who treat their illnesses with full doses of sodium thiosulfate pentahydrate and alpha ketoglutaric acid, and who do not take the Vital B12 injections. The author does not take the Vital B12 injections, and he has acquired both the sublingual methylcobalamin 5,000 mcg tablets and the sublingual hydroxocobalamin 5,000 mcg tablets per Amazon. He usually takes the methylcobalamin tablets because he has found them to be much less expensive than the hydroxocobalamin tablets.

Chapter Two
Testimonials

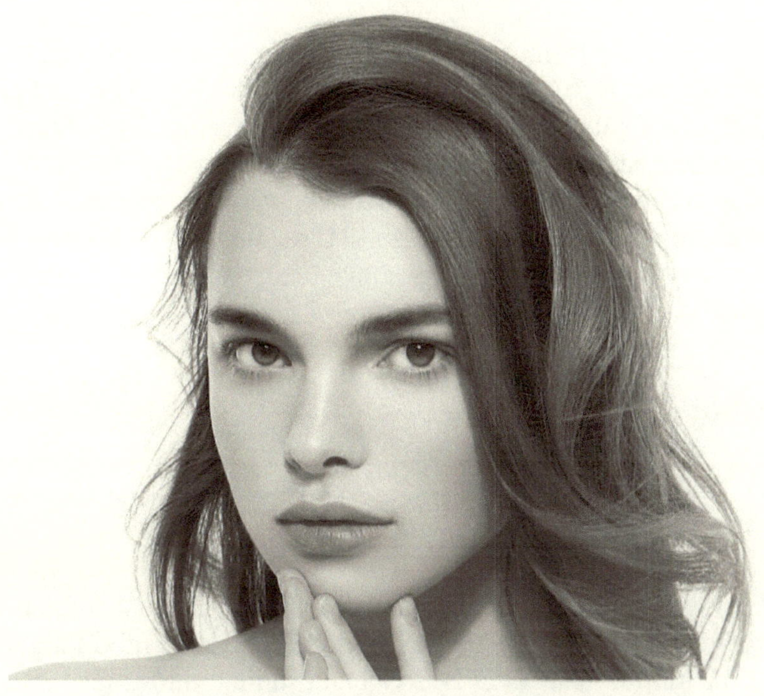

<u>A Female Fibromyalgia Patient Who is an Author</u>:

Before beginning treatment, my best days were wracked with pain and inability to focus or accomplish the simplest things. I don't know how many days I cursed by body and its inability to perform simple tasks. Since beginning treatment, my quality of life has improved on levels I never thought were possible. The fibro fog, which makes it difficult to focus, has also lessened to the point that I rarely notice it. I've begun losing weight since I am now able to be more active. This treatment has changed my life for the better. Less pain, less fog, no more crying jags because of the things I couldn't do. If you suffer from fibro, I urge you to try the treatment. I take the full treatment and I haven't felt this good in over 15 years!

* * * * * * *

<u>A Retired Army Veteran with Diabetes and Rheumatoid Arthritis</u>:

Approximately 18 months ago I was having trouble keeping my blood sugar and HgbA1C in proper balance. I wished to control my blood readings without the use of insulin. My average daily blood sugar reading had climbed higher than 126 and my HgbA1C was hovering around 7.0. I began treatment. Now my average daily blood sugar reading is 98 and my last HgbA1C reading was 5.3. I have also come off my methotrexate for RA since taking a Vital B12 shot daily.

Thank you for your help.

A true convert.

* * * * * * *

<u>A Lady with Multiple Sclerosis Whose Husband has
Rheumatoid Arthritis</u>:

Thank you so much for prescribing Vital B12 Gel and sodium thiosulfate for me. As you know, I have MS and have mild fatigue from time to time. The Vital B12 Gel and sodium thiosulfate have helped so much, my entire body and mind just feel better. It has completely taken care of my fatigue. I have been using it about 15 months and will continue. Also my husband has RA and is using sodium thiosulfate. He has been amazed in the difference in his ankle and knee movement immediately after starting the therapy.

Thank you so much.

* * * * * * *

<u>A Lady with Fibromyalgia at Age 70</u>:

When we lived in Iowa I went to a Rheumatologist to, I thought, be diagnosed as to what kind of arthritis I had. My whole body ached all the way to my fingertips. After the doctor examined me, he said that I didn't have rheumatoid arthritis. He said I had a tad bit of osteoarthritis but what I did have was fibromyalgia and he didn't need to see me again! That had become a new word in my vocabulary! I found that this was something I had to live with, but what would help is if I didn't over do my daily tasks. That is hard to do. My brain was fuzzy and I had a hard time focusing on tasks that had to be done. I attributed it to early onset of old age! But I was glad this wasn't something that was terminal.

You prescribed the Vital B12 and recommended other supplements. Before I left the office I was given my first Vital B12 shot. All I could say was "Wow!" Almost instantly I experienced something that I can best describe like when the sun is behind the cloud and all of a sudden the cloud goes away and the sun shines. I felt like a totally new person! It was unbelievable. I even wondered if it was my imagination! But we bought the Vital B12 and other supplements at the compounding pharmacy before we returned home. I give myself a Vital B12 shot every third day and I can tell you that I feel like a different person! Instead of moving slowly when I go from place to place in our home I find myself moving more rapidly and I am getting more things accomplished. I can think more clearly. I can read and absorb what I read. Before I would read a paragraph and at the end of the paragraph I wondered what I had read! As I look back, I am convinced that I was suffering from Fibromyalgia long before I was diagnosed.

I hope this gives you some indication as to how your discovery has changed my life.

* * * * * * *

A Male in his Fifties with Fibromyalgia:

When I am asked what it's like to have fibromyalgia, I describe it as similar to having a never-ending low-grade influenza. The feverishness is there along with joint pain and muscle aches. But, within an hour after receiving the first Vital B12 injection, the body aches were all but gone. The pain was not debilitating, but was always there, even affecting my sleep. I like to think of myself as an upbeat, cheery person but had to admit the fact that being in pain 24-7 is no fun! So, relieving the pain has improved my sleep and mood, as well. I also seem to have more stamina and am considering resuming a daily jogging routine.

* * * * * * *

A Female with Chronic Fatigue and Fibromyalgia:

I am a 32 year-old Nurse Practitioner. I have suffered from Chronic Fatigue since childhood and Fibromyalgia since my 20s. I had been on some more conventional medications for the Fibromyalgia. Many I was unable to tolerate and those that I could tolerate were becoming much less effective. I have taken various dosing regimens of the Vital B12 and although all helped the best treatment for me has been a daily injection.

I also took the Alpha Ketoglutaric Acid for months after starting the treatment and this also helped. However, I found that after months of daily injections of B12 I no longer needed the AKG acid.

I have noticed less fatigue and decreased pain. In addition to the chronic all over flu-like aching, it had gotten to the point that I also had intermittent and migrating joint pain and all 4 of my extremities (arms, legs) were numb. They always felt like pins and needles—like when your foot goes to sleep. The joint pain is almost completely resolved, I only have a few patches of numbness now and on a typical day the all over aching has decreased to a mild annoyance. I now have the energy to go to work and go home and play with my son and enjoy my husband's company. Sadly before starting the treatment all I felt like doing was sitting around on the couch by the time I got home.

I consider it a blessing that my eyes have been opened to this treatment.

* * * * * * *

<u>A Professional Business Editor and Certified Quality Auditor with Chronic Fatigue Syndrome (Female)</u>:

I struggled with fatigue for years, since the mid-1990s. Back then, there wasn't a name for what is now known as chronic fatigue syndrome. So, even though I was only in my mid-thirties, I attributed the fatigue to "getting older." Several years ago I was prescribed a fatigue-blocking medication (Nuvigil) that enabled me to work (technical editor), but I still felt tired all the time. The medication just made the fatigue manageable (barely).

Then I was diagnosed as likely having cyanide sensitivity syndrome. I was told that if I had it, the recommended treatment would make me feel better and that if I didn't have it, the treatment would do no harm. I'd been tired all the time for so long that I would try anything that might help, no matter how unusual it sounded. So, I tried it, and this *treatment actually <u>helped</u>*. It didn't completely fix the problem, but it helped in a way that nothing else had. I felt better—less tired, less mentally "fuzzy."

I was given a prescription for compounded B12 shots, with the recommendation that I take sodium thiosulfate in water every two hours, and I was provided with a short list of over-the-counter supplements to be taken daily. Based on the results, there's no question that I have cyanide sensitivity syndrome. For example, I take sodium thiosulfate in water every two hours, as recommended, and I can tell when the two hours are almost up because I can feel it wearing off and the fatigue starting to come back.

After three years, I returned to the doctor who diagnosed me with cyanide sensitivity syndrome. The doctor recommended adding Alpha Ketoglutaric Acid three times a day, taken in the powder form in water (rather than in capsules). I tried it, and the results were startling. *I felt normal for the first time in years. I felt alert and like I had a normal energy level.* I immediately added Alpha Ketoglutaric Acid powder to my daily routine, and I've been taking it regularly ever since. I must add that the Alpha Ketoglutaric Acid, even combined with the rest of the treatment regime, is not a miracle cure. I wish it was, but I've learned that if I push the physical/mental envelope too hard, the chronic fatigue will override the positive effect of any treatment.

In summary, it's hard to find words to describe the difference that the treatment has made in my life without sounding over the top. It's my understanding that the recommended treatment regime is not yet accepted by the mainstream medical profession. However, I hope that my personal account and those from others like me will help it gain acceptance. The treatment might be considered off-normal or unorthodox, but *it works*, and that's what really matters. In closing, the treatment does no harm, and God knows, I'm living proof of how much the treatment helps when the diagnosis is on target.

<u>Chapter Three</u>
CFS/ME/SEID
Chronic Fatigue Syndrome
Myalgic Encephalomyelitis
Systemic Exertional Intolerance Disease

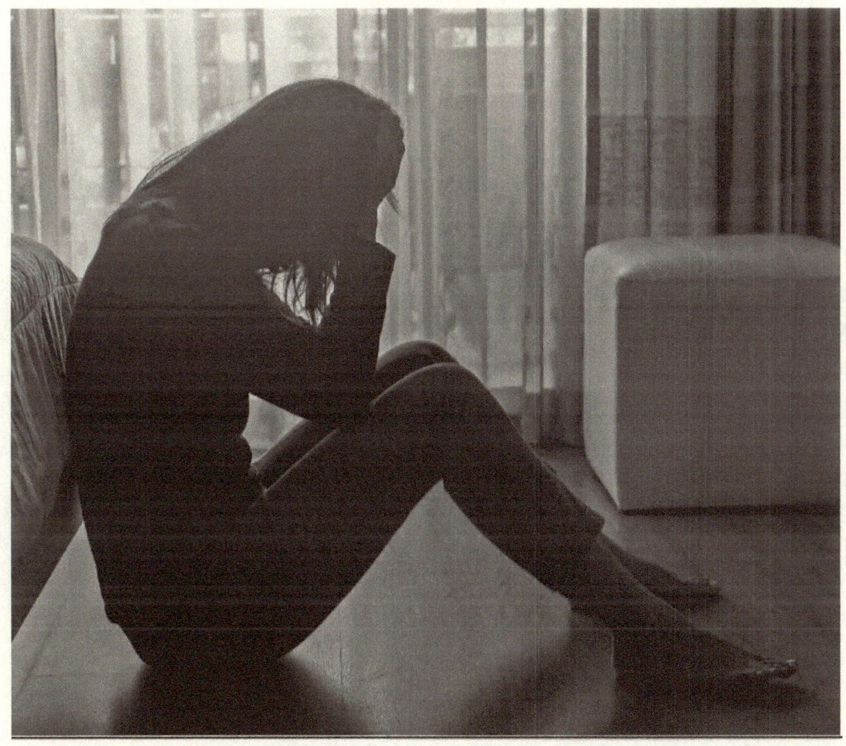

    Although the author now considers environmental cyanide intoxication to be his specialty; in 1981, the existence of such an entity was totally new to him. Furthermore, to the best of the author's memory, it was years thereafter before he ever heard the phrase, *chronic*

fatigue syndrome. Therefore, he believes that he can make an unbiased comparison between the symptoms of environmental cyanide intoxication and those of chronic fatigue syndrome by restating data from a report that he wrote in 1982—before ever hearing of *chronic fatigue syndrome* (CFS). Chronic fatigue syndrome later obtained the name, *myalgic encephalomyelitis* (ME), and has more recently been given the denotation, *systemic exertional intolerance disease* (SEID).

First, for comparison, the following web address may be opened to find ten symptoms of chronic fatigue syndrome, namely *weakness, pain, getting sick, difficulty sleeping, cognitive impairment, tingling, dizziness, sensitivity to stimuli, cannot stand for long,* and *stomach problems*:

https://10faq.com/health/chronic-fatigue-syndrome-symptoms/?utm_source=bing&utm_medium=cpc&utm_campaign=USA%20-%20Chronic%20Fatigue%20Syndrome%20-%20Desktop&utm_term=chronic%20fatigue%20syndrome%20symptoms&utm_content=Chronic%20Fatigue%20Syndrome%20Symptoms

And then, note the symptoms appearing in the following paragraphs that were written by the author after acquiring positive testing for cyanide and/or thiocyanate in about eighty patients who were suffering from environmental cyanide intoxication in the early 1980s. The paragraphs are copied, in quotes, word for word, as penned by the author in an article he wrote in 1982, entitled, *Metropolitan Effects of Environmental Cyanide* [1]:

"Tiredness and depression are probably most universal of the symptoms my patients experience. Increased time in bed, restless sleep, lack of motivation, and apathetic withdrawal depict aspects of the depression."

"Athletic and mental abilities are also altered in affected patients. These impairments come and go, but a generalized deterioration occurs during the course of recurring episodes of illness. In a few instances, episodes of relief seem rarer than those of illness. Decreased exercise tolerance, lower grades in school, forgetfulness, and inability to concentrate are also noteworthy features in these patients."

"Jacobs [2] mentions several other symptoms of chronic cyanide exposure which are very prevalent in the patients I see, namely weakness, nausea, muscle cramps, loss of appetite, and psychoses. Another author reports pallor, vertigo, indigestion, and breathlessness [3], which are also common among my patients. He further states that in some patients the picture may be that of a mental illness. I have noted that a remarkable number of patients have been advised to see psychologists or psychiatrists prior to their diagnosis of cyanide poisoning."

"Another patient, again a nonsmoker, had a urine thiocyanate level of 15.4 mg/L on the fourth day after hospitalization for an attack of dizziness. He first became ill on a Wednesday and was hospitalized the following Friday. On that same Wednesday, a woman who lived across the street from this man also became ill, and died the following Friday. Her symptoms, from what I was told, included dizziness, shortness of breath, and an elevated temperature. Several patients I have treated for acute cyanide poisoning had mildly elevated temperatures, …"

"The majority of patients I am treating report significant relief from headaches using sodium thiosulfate alone."

Although not plainly stated in the above sentences that were written in 1982, the author has definitely associated cyanide sensitivity with decreased immune function and getting sick more often. The entire report, entitled, *Metropolitan Effects of Environmental Cyanide,* is rather lengthy; but for anyone interested, it is included in the novel entitled, *A Breath of Cyanide,* by Timothy Swiss. Much of the material in *A Breath of Cyanide* was written in the 1980s, including the following sentences which are presented in quotes and written in italics. These sentences describe the very first patient who the author diagnosed with cyanide intoxication:

"He was actually suffering a number of symptoms, but the strangest were painful sensations in his in his hands and fingers. There was no notable joint inflammation, just unexplained pain and tingling. At first I explored conventional etiologies: arthritis, gout, vitamin deficiency, etc. Nothing turned up positive. Finally I decided to stop retracing

tests done by prior physicians and move to new ground. I asked John what he was exposed to at work."

The author believes that airborne cyanide is likely the most common cause of ME (myalgic encephomyelitis), and following is a comparative list of published findings and symptoms comparing those of cyanide intoxication to those symptoms of ME. The author added the words, *oxygen is important for the immune system to work properly*. These words were added in italics and enclosed in parentheses, and they were included by the author as a description of one mechanism by which cyanide may contribute to episodes of illness, including sore throat and tender lymph nodes.

<u>Cyanide</u>	<u>CFS/ME (Myalgic Encephalomyelitis)</u>
1. general weakness	1.) muscle weakness
2. confusion	2.) cognitive impairment
3. bizarre behavior	3.) personality change
4. excessive sleepiness	4.) unrefreshing sleep
5. coma	5.) coma-like experiences
6. shortness of breath	6.) shortness of breath
7. headache	7.) headaches, either new or worsening
8. dizziness	8.) dizziness is common
9. vomiting	9.) digestive issues
10. abdominal pain	10.) irritable bowel syndrome
11. seizures	11.) seizures
12. lethargy	12.) fatigue

13. elevated lactic acid	13.) exercise increases lactate accumulation
14. anxiety	14.) anxiety
15. chest pain	15.) chest pain
16. joint and muscle aches and pains	16.) joint pain, muscle pain and aches
17. cyanide blocks the body's ability to use oxygen	17.) sore throat and tender lymph nodes (*oxygen is important for the immune system to work properly*)
18. tachycardia and abnormal ECG	18.) tachycardia and abnormal ECG
19. perspiration	19.) chills and night sweats

<u>How Airborne Cyanide May Cause the Inflammation of Brain and Nerve Tissue Seen in Myalgic Encephalomyelitis</u>

The brain and nerve tissues are sensitive to hypoxia, with the brain being the most sensitive organ in the body to lack of oxygen. One form of hypoxia is histotoxic hypoxia, with cyanide being a prime example of an agent that causes histotoxic hypoxia. Hypoxia in neuronal tissue, in turn, causes inflammation. Thus, the encephalomyelitis noted in ME is consistent with cyanide being the most common underlying cause of ME.

* * * * * * *

Sometime prior to May 6, 1992, the author received a phone call at work from a researcher in Ann Arbor, Michigan. The researcher spoke with him for almost an hour before the author excused himself to return to his duties as an occupational physician. This researcher had the hypothesis that chronic fatigue syndrome results from viral interference with the physiologic metabolism of cyanide. He pointed out that mitochondrial and neurologic abnormalities shown in chronic fatigue syndrome are consistent with effects of cyanide. The author assured the researcher that he might be pursuing one of the most important medical discoveries of the century; and the author also pointed out that lactic acidosis, fatigue, mental impedance, exercise intolerance, and basically the entire gamut of symptoms attributed to chronic fatigue syndrome are consistent with cyanide intoxication. The author wants to clarify, to the reader, that he does not believe that any virus has to be involved for persons to become sensitive to cyanide, but he would certainly be open-minded to the possibility that a viral infection may sometimes be a trigger for an individual to develop cyanide sensitivity.

References:

1.) Sentences from 1982 article: *Metropolitan Effects of Environmental Cyanide*—written per the author in Houston, Texas during his initial treatment of patients suffering illness from sensitivity to airborne cyanide. The article has now been published, as of July 18, 2020, in the book entitled, *A Breath of Cyanide,* by Timothy Swiss.
2.) M.B. Jacobs. "*Analytical Toxicology of Industrial Inorganic Poisons*", "Wiley Interscience Mag": 721-741 (1967).
3.) C.J. Polson and R.N. Tattersall. *Clinical Toxicology*, published by J.B. Lippincott Company in North America, and by Pitman Medical Publishing Company Ltd in Great Britain, pp. 132-155 (1975).

Chapter Four
Fibromyalgia

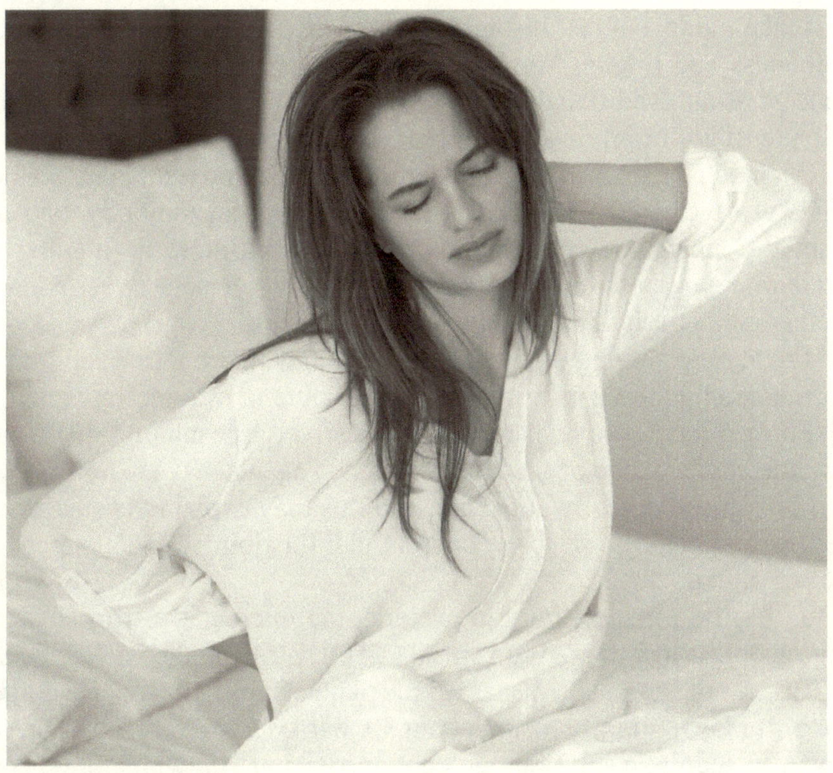

In 1982, a microallergist in Houston, Dr. William Hitt, tested 43 persons (*mostly nonsmokers*) who were suspected of or diagnosed with cyanide intoxication resulting from airborne cyanide pollution. Dr. William M. Hitt had a Ph.D. in Microbiology and Applied Biology from a number of schools. He finished at Johns Hopkins.

Dr. Hitt found that 25 (58%) of these persons tested positive for immunological sensitivity to cyanide, whereas only one of 200 control patients tested positive. As the primary physician treating most of these patients, the author came to recognize that the more common symptoms of cyanide intoxication included such things as fatigue, depression, headache, memory problems, decreased resistance to infections, restless sleep, weakness, muscle cramps, forgetfulness, inability to concentrate, exercise intolerance, muscle aches, and joint pain. Comparatively, the National Fibromyalgia Research Association listed symptoms occurring in 40% or more of fibromyalgia patients as muscular pains, fatigue, insomnia, joint pains, headaches, restless legs, numbness and tingling, impaired memory, leg cramps, and impaired concentration. Additionally, nervousness was reported to occur in 32% of patients with fibromyalgia and major depression in 20%.

Cyanide is a small molecule that may not be antigenic, but cyanide binds to several enzymes and other entities within the body, and the resultant molecules may be antigenic. In addition to binding to cytochrome oxidase, cyanide reportedly binds to catalase, peroxidase, methemoglobin, hydroxocobalamin, phosphatase, tyrosinase, ascorbic acid oxidase, xanthine oxidase, and succinic dehydrogenase; and it has been noted that these reactions may contribute to cyanide's toxicity [1, 2]. Furthermore, cyanide is reportedly a carboxylase inhibitor [3]. Thus, cyanide bound to one of the aforementioned agents may create an entity that is immunologically antigenic; and this may explain the significant degree of aching muscles and/or painful joints encountered in fibromyalgia.

In testing for sensitivity to cyanide, the microallergist in Houston spun blood at low to medium speed (1,500 rpm) and then collected the buffy layer of serum and discarded the platelets from the top. He diluted the buffy layer slightly, using about six parts serum to one part sterile water, to acquire a solution that contained about 100 white blood cells per field using 450X magnification plus a 15X viewing lens. Using meticulously cleaned glassware and equipment, he prepared antigen jelly slides using Vaseline petroleum jelly as an inert base. Generally, twenty milligrams of an antigen to be tested were mixed in 20 milliliters of water and allowed to sit overnight. (*Note: the author has no record of how the antigen that was used in testing patients for immunological sensitivity to cyanide was prepared. It would seem logical, though, to first obtain a sample of proteins from the individual who is being tested, such as from blood, urine, and buccal smears; and to then add some cyanide to these proteins and gently mix the cyanide with the proteins; and to then place twenty milligrams of the mixture of cyanide and proteins into twenty milliliters of water and permit this final mixture to sit overnight in an airtight container at about 98.6 degrees Fahrenheit. Sitting overnight should give the cyanide time to bind to receptor sites on the protein molecules, thus forming antigens to which an individual may be immunologically sensitive. This, then, would provide the antigenic solution for testing.*) About 2.5 drops of this antigenic solution were placed on a ring of jelly that was about 1 cm in diameter.

One large drop of WBCs was added to each antigen-jelly slide. On control slides, the WBCs would not disrupt for about 2 to 3 hours; whereas, on slides where sensitivity was determined to exist, cells would disrupt in about thirty minutes. The speed and degree of disruption of the white blood cells was observed, and the degree of sensitivity was determined from such observation. Although some of the persons determined to be suffering from cyanide intoxication did not show immunological sensitivity to cyanide at all (*and may have been suffering due to metabolic inadequacies rather than immunological sensitivity*); other persons, some of whom were notably ill, did show marked immunological sensitivity.

The author definitely believes that persons who develop immunological sensitivity to cyanide may also suffer from cyanide intoxication secondary to impaired ability to metabolize cyanide, such as may be found in chronic fatigue syndrome. Treatment of patients with cyanide intoxication who are immunologically sensitive to cyanide, though, may prove more challenging than treating patients with cyanide intoxication who are not immunologically sensitive to cyanide; and such treatment may require very consistent and thorough maintenance doses of the recommended antidotes. With fibromyalgia, the author has generally recommended 0.5 cc of the Vital B12 injected daily, and this may be supplemented with the other treatments. The Vital B12 and other treatments are described in detail in the first chapter of this book.

References:

1.) Ardelt BK, Borowitz JL, Isom GE. Brain lipid peroxidation and antioxidant protectant mechanisms following acute cyanide intoxication. Toxicology 56:147-154, 1989.

2.) Rieders F. Noxious gases and vapors I: Carbon monoxide, cyanides, methemoglobin, and sulfhemoglobin. In: DePalma JR, ed. Drill's pharmacology in medicine, 4th ed. New York, NY: McGraw-Hill Book Company, 1180-1205, 1971.

3.) De Metz M, Soute BAM, Hemker HC, Vermeer C. The inhibition of Vitamin K-Dependent Carboxylase by Cyanide. FEBS Lett 137(2):253-256, January 1982.

Chapter Five
Autism

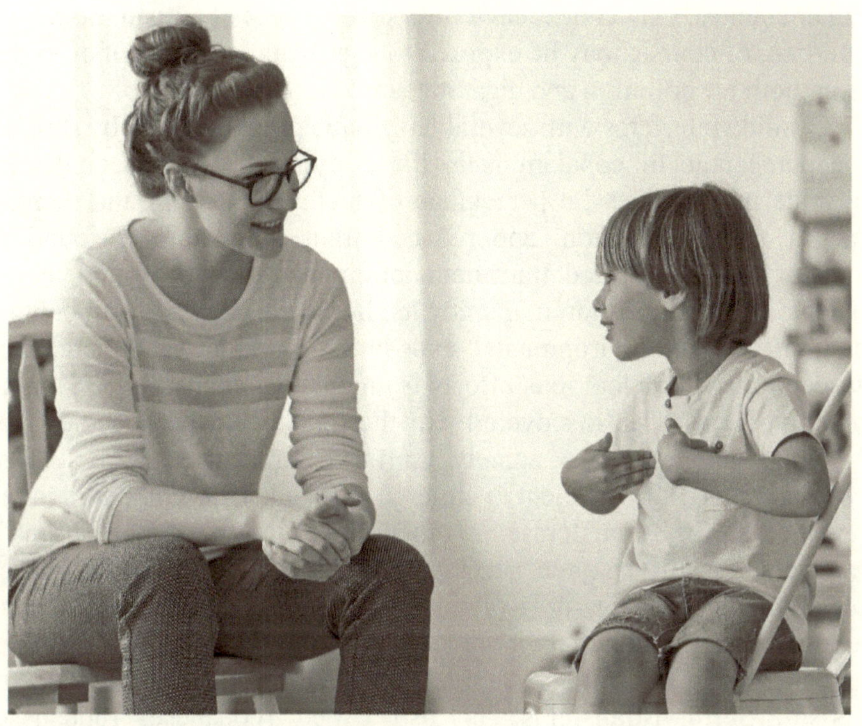

A study published November 5, 2018 reports that exposure to outdoor air pollution increases the incidence of autism by up to 78% [1]. Cyanide inhibits reactions in which pyridoxal phosphate functions as a coenzyme (*a coenzyme is a nonprotein, organic compound that is necessary for the functioning of an enzyme; and note that pyridoxal phosphate, or vitamin B6, is sometimes referred to as a cofactor rather than as a coenzyme*); and deficiency of pyridoxal phosphate—which may be expected to yield similar results to inhibition of pyridoxal phosphate—results in a decrease in the neurotransmitters serotonin and GABA [2, 3, 4]. Cyanide may inhibit a child's normal spike of serotonin during late pregnancy and early childhood and result in decreased synaptic formation in the brain, thus contributing to autism [5, 6, 7]. Such suppression of brain development may be most severe where cyanide exposure is constant, such as in regions with high levels of air pollution; and this may result in more severe types of autism. Intermittent exposure to cyanide, such as when a mother or father smokes, may contribute to less severe types of autism. Some children, of course, may be exposed to significant amounts of cyanide from both air pollution and cigarette smoke.

Cyanide interferes with several enzymatic processes, and by shifting the percentage of cobalamins in the body toward cyanocobalamin, cyanide may reduce the percentage of methylcobalamin and thereby inhibit transmethylation; and reduced transmethylation is found in autism [8, 9]. Reduced transmethylation may also be found in the parents of autistic children, thereby lending evidence to autism being a combination of environmental exposure to cyanide and hereditary susceptibility to deleterious effects from cyanide exposure [8, 9]. And notably, it has been discovered that the major enzyme necessary for metabolizing cyanide, namely sulfuryl-transferase (*also called rhodanese, etc.*), is deficient in children with autism as compared to the level of sulfuryl-transferase in other children [10]. Since sulfuryl-transferase is the enzyme necessary for the body's major means of metabolizing cyanide, it is obvious that lack of sulfuryl-transferase activity leaves individuals more susceptible to the effects of cyanide; and therefore, this finding supports cyanide as a causative agent in autism. Sulfuryl-transferase is also called rhodanese, rhodanase, thiosulfate sulfurtransferase, thiosulfate cyanide transsulfurase, and thiosulfate thiotransferase. Higher levels of thiocyanate found in some autistic children would not be expected from reduced rhodanese activity, and may simply indicate that those children experience exposure to higher quantities of cyanide than other children; and note that, if the autistic children with higher quantities of thiocyanate metabolize cyanide at a slower rate than other children, such reduced efficiency in metabolizing cyanide would increase their vulnerability to deleterious effects from cyanide; and thus, the increased level of thiocyanate in some autistic children is not inconsistent with cyanide as the causative agent for autism. Furthermore, an inherent decreased rate of metabolizing cyanide in autistic children would indicate that those children may suffer toxic symptoms from airborne cyanide exposure and may benefit from antidotes for cyanide.

Foods rich in sulfur would be expected to aid the body's ability to detoxify cyanide to thiocyanate; and notably, the maternal intake of nuts, eggs, and/or salmon during pregnancy, all being high in sulfur content, is associated with a reduced incidence of autism [11, 12]. The intake of nuts is also found to reduce the incidence of diabetes [13]; and as with autism, there is a strong link between air pollution and diabetes [14]. The occurrence of diabetes is increased in autistic adults, and there is increased autism in the children of diabetic mothers, and there is increased insulin resistance in both diabetes and autism [15]. Cyanide causes production of nitric oxide that inhibits methionine synthase, and decreased activity of methionine synthase is found in autism [16]. Treating older autistic children and adults with antidotes for cyanide poisoning—such as hydroxocobalamin, methylcobalamin, vitamin B6, alpha ketoglutaric acid, and sodium thiosulfate pentahydrate—may not reverse the lack of synaptic formation, but will likely improve function in those children and adults. Such treatment may prevent autism if given to pregnant mothers, infants, and younger children.

Methylcobalamin appears to be especially important in treating autism [17], and it should be included in any treatment regimen for autism. The author recommends the subcutaneous or intramuscular injection of a mixture of 15 milligrams per cc of methylcobalamin and 10 milligrams per cc of hydroxocobalamin, for a total of 25 milligrams of vitamin B12 per cc, given as a one cc dose of 25 milligrams at least every three days. (*Note: the Vital B12, which is described in chapter one of this book, may also be used for persons with autism. Vital B12 is a mixture of 12.5 milligrams per cc of hydroxocobalamin and 12.5 milligrams per cc of methylcobalamin, for a total vitamin B12 concentration of 25 milligrams per cc*). The author recommends _avoiding_ cyanocobalamin as a source of vitamin B12. Cyanocobalamin is a synthetic form of vitamin B12 that is not natural to the body, and that contains a cyanide molecule; and cyanocobalamin is what hydroxocobalamin is converted to when it serves as an antidote for cyanide poisoning [18]. In the event that the FDA ever makes injectable methylcobalamin illegal, which would be tragic, then the author would recommend supplementing injectable hydroxocobalamin with sublingual methylcobalamin.

And finally, in regard to autism, be sure and read the next to last paragraph in chapter six of this book, the chapter entitled, *Diabetes*.

<u>References</u>:

1.) ScienceDaily, *Air pollution linked to autism*, Monash University, November 5, 2018—internet address: https://www.sciencedaily.com/releases/2018/11/18110510541 4.htm   and also see: https://www.scientificamerican.com/article/autism-risk-linked-to-particulate-air-pollution/

2.) Isom GE, Liu DHW, Way JL. *Effect of Sublethal Doses of Cyanide on Glucose Catabolism*. Biochem Pharmacol 24(8):871-5, 1975.

3.) Dakshinamurti K, LeBlancq WD, Herchi R, Haulicek V. *Brain monoamines of pyridoxine-deficient growing rats*. Exp. Brain Res. 26:355-66, 1976.

4.) Dakshinamurti K, Paulose CS, Siow YL. *Neurobiology of pyridoxine*. In: Reynolds RD, Leklem JE. Vitamin B-6: Its Role in Health and Disease. New York: Alan R. Liss, Inc., pp. 99-121, 1985.

5.) <u>Int Rev Neurobiol.</u> 2004;59:111-74, *Serotonin and brain development*, <u>Sodhi MS</u>[1], <u>Sanders-Bush E</u>

6.) <u>Neuroscience. 2017 Feb 7; 342: 212–231</u>, Published online 2016 Feb 22. Doi: 10.1016/j.neuroscience.2016.02.037, *DEVELOPMENTAL CHANGES IN SEROTONIN SIGNALING: IMPLICATIONS FOR EARLY BRAIN FUNCTION, BEHAVIOR AND ADAPTATION*, <u>S. BRUMMELTE</u>,[a,*] <u>E. MC GLANAGHY</u>,[b,c] <u>A. BONNIN</u>,[d] and <u>T. F. OBERLANDER</u>—internet address: https://www.ncbi.nlm.nih.gov/pmc/articles/PMC5310545/

7.) The DANA Foundation, *Cerebrum, timely and provocative articles on neuroscience*, Tuesday, August 6, 2006, Bringing the Brain of the Child with Autism Back on Track, Diane C. Chugani, Ph.D, and Kayt Sukel—internet address: http://www.dana.org/Cerebrum/2006/Bringing_the_Brain_of_t he_Child_with_Autism_Back_on_Track/

8.) J Autism Dev Disord. 2008 Nov; 38(10): 1966–1975., Published online 2008 May 30. doi: 10.1007/s10803-008-0591-5, *Abnormal transmethylation/transsulfuration metabolism and DNA hypomethylation among parents of children with autism,* S. Jill James,[a] Stepan Melnyk,[a] Stefanie Jernigan,[a] Amanda Hubanks,[a] Shannon Rose,[a] and David W. Gaylor—internet address: https://www.ncbi.nlm.nih.gov/pmc/articles/PMC2584168/

9.) AUTISM AND CHILDREN WHO CANNOT DETOXIFY, American Journal of Clinical Nutrition 2004 80 (December):1611-1617. *Metabolic biomarkers of increased oxidative stress and impaired methylation capacity in children with autism.* S Jill James, Paul Cutler, Stepan Melnyk, Stefanie Jernigan, Laurette Janak, David W Gaylor and James A Neubrander—internet address: https://www.cfwellness.com/autism-and-children-who-cannot-detoxify/

10.) LIVEJOURNAL, *Rhodanese problems in autism: how to recognize and possibly prevent*-Alobar   Grewalker: Magickai Record (aka Frater PVN, LA-BAJ-AL), October 28th, 2010—internet address: https://alobar.livejournal.com/4175904.html#/4175904.html

11.) See internet address: https://www.pregnancymagazine.com/pregnancy/pregnancy-health/your-pregnancy-diet-and-autism

12.) See internet address: https://www.thehealthyhomeeconomist.com/autism-risk-significantly-reduced-with-preconception-nutrition/

13.) See internet address: https://www.diabeticsweekly.com/eating-nuts-prevent-type-ii-diabetes/

14.) ScienceDaily, *Air pollution contributes significantly to diabetes globally. Even low pollution levels can pose health risk.* June 30, 2018. Washington University in St. Louis. New research links outdoor air pollution – even at levels deemed safe – to an increased risk of diabetes globally, according to a new study. The findings raise the possibility that reducing pollution may lead to a drop in diabetes cases in heavily polluted countries such as India and less polluted ones such as the United States. See internet address: https://www.sciencedaily.com/releases/2018/06/180630153740.htm

15.) ScienceDaily; *Common link suggested between autism and diabetes*: Study implicates hyperinsulinemia in increased incidence of autism; October 19, 2011, Rice University. Internet address: https://www.sciencedaily.com/releases/2011/10/111019184622.htm

16.) See internet addresses: https://drbratt.com/treatment-methylation-deficits-autism-spectrum-disorder/   and: https://www.ncbi.nlm.nih.gov/pubmed/11371572   and: https://www.ncbi.nlm.nih.gov/pubmed/8613912   and: http://jpet.aspetjournals.org/content/285/1/236.short

17.) J Child Adolesc Psychopharmacol. 2016 Nov;26(9):774-783. Epub 2016 Feb 18. *Randomized, Placebo-Controlled Trial of Methyl B12 for Children with Autism*. Hendren RL, James SJ, Widjaja F, Lawton B, Rosenblatt A, Bent S. See internet address: https://www.ncbi.nlm.nih.gov/pubmed/26889605

18.) See internet address: http://epmonthly.com/article/hydroxocobalamin-turning-cyanide-into-vitamin-b12/

Chapter Six
Diabetes

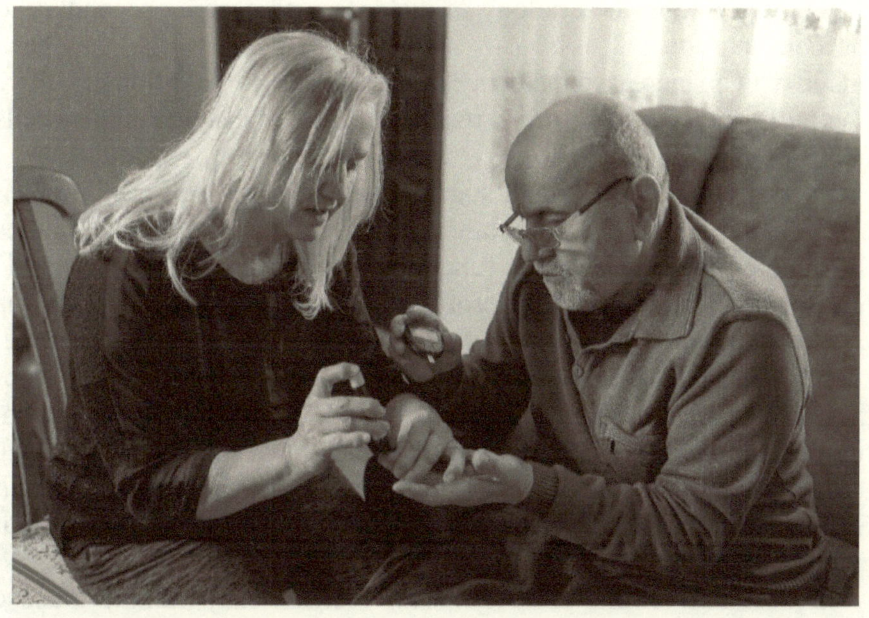

(*Note: in regard to diabetes, be sure and read the third paragraph in Chapter 5, the chapter on autism. That paragraph refers to a publication from June of 2018 that reports a strong link between air pollution and diabetes. This 2018 publication is listed as reference number fourteen at the end of chapter 5.)

Sulfur-containing amino acids are known to assist the body in detoxifying cyanide, and amino acid supplementation with cysteine, methionine, and taurine has been proffered as adjuvant therapy in the treatment of diabetes [1]. Also of note, intake of either cysteine or taurine is reported to reduce homocysteine levels [1]. Increased homocysteine levels are associated with heart disease, which is prevalent in diabetics, and the author recommends taking vitamins B6, B12, and folic acid (B9) along with any sulfur-containing amino acid supplementation. Vitamins B6, B12, and folic acid are important in lowering homocysteine levels, and instructions on how to dose these three vitamins are given in chapter one of this book.

The author's research indicates that airborne cyanide is indigenous to modern, industrialized society, and that it is present in the atmospheres of cities and towns around the world [2]. Chemical toxins may play a role in the etiology of diabetes, and cyanide secondary to the consumption of cassava (*a dietary source of cyanide*) has been linked with an increased incidence of diabetes [3, 4]. Additionally, there is experimental evidence of a direct toxic effect of cyanide on beta cells in the pancreas [3].

Cyanide may alter normal sugar metabolism through inhibition of carboxylase, inhibition of amylase synthesis, and inhibition of reactions in which pyridoxal phosphate functions as a coenzyme [5, 6]. Cyanide is also noted to promote anaerobic metabolism and to decrease the concentration of ATP [1, 6]. Notably, glucose is the only fuel that will supply energy to skeletal muscle under anaerobic conditions [7]. For these reasons, and for other reasons that will be addressed further on, the development and progression of diabetes, as well as the reactive hypoglycemia that sometimes heralds the onset of diabetes, may result from individual sensitivity and/or vulnerability to environmental cyanide.

In addition to the previous data, cyanide may inhibit glucose tolerance factor (GTF) by binding to the metallic cofactor (*a cofactor is a substance that is necessary for the activity of an enzyme*), namely chromium [8]. As early as 1977, it was noted that diabetics often exhibit altered chromium metabolism, but the precise relation of this metal to diabetes remained uncertain [9]. More recent information from the Agency for Toxic Substances and Disease Registry in Atlanta states that chromium III plays a role in maintaining normal metabolism of glucose, fat, and cholesterol [10]. It goes on to state that chromium III appears to potentiate insulin action, probably in the form of glucose tolerance factor; and that chromium deficiency is characterized by glucose intolerance, glycosuria, hypercholesterolemia, decreased longevity, decreased sperm counts, and impaired fertility [10]. In one patient receiving total parental nutrition, a peripheral neuropathy was corrected after chromium supplementation [10]. Thus, the binding of cyanide to chromium in glucose tolerance factor may inhibit the enzymatic activity of that agent and contribute to insulin resistance. Such insulin resistance may contribute to increased production of glucose by the liver, and to decreased uptake of glucose by tissues such as muscle and fat [11].

In time, the toxicity of cyanide to beta cells may result in diabetes through the gradual destruction of those cells. Since cyanide causes histotoxic hypoxia, it is reasonable to assume that there may be some associated inflammation, and that the inflammation may play a role in the destruction of beta cells. It has been estimated that 25% to 80% of beta cells within an individual's pancreas have been destroyed prior to that individual's onset of diabetes. Steps to prevent diabetes, or stop the progression of diabetes, may be achieved through the use of agents such as hydroxocobalamin (*a form of vitamin B12*), sodium thiosulfate pentahydrate, alpha-ketoglutaric acid [12], and chromium picolinate. The author recommends 200 mcg of chromium picolinate twice daily, one dose each morning and one dose each evening, for a total of 400 mcg per day. Larger doses may be appropriate if recommended by an individual's private physician. Cinnamon also appears to be of notable benefit in regard to diabetes.

A factor associated with Type 1 Diabetes is the formation of autoantibodies to one or more of three agents: insulin, 65-kd glutamic acid decarboxylase, and tyrosine phosphatases [13]. In 1982, a microallergist in Houston tested 43 persons (*mostly nonsmokers*) who were suspected of or diagnosed with cyanide intoxication, and found that 25 (58%) tested positive for immunological sensitivity to cyanide, whereas only one of 200 control patients tested positive. The scale used by the microallergist to grade the degree of sensitivity was 0, +, ++, or +++; and persons reportedly sensitive to cyanide received grades ranging from + to +++, indicating that some of them were very sensitive to cyanide immunologically. Since cyanide is a very small molecule consisting of only one carbon atom and one nitrogen atom, it appears very unlikely to be an antigen. However, a substance formed in vivo by the union of cyanide with a more complex molecule may be antigenic, in which case cyanide is functioning as a hapten. A hapten is a small molecule that can combine to a larger molecule, such as a protein, and form a resultant molecule that may induce an autoimmune or allergic reaction.

In addition to binding to cytochrome oxidase, cyanide reportedly binds to catalase, peroxidase, methemoglobin, hydroxocobalamin, phosphatase, tyrosinase, ascorbic acid oxidase, xanthine oxidase, and succinic dehydrogenase; and it has been noted that these reactions may contribute to cyanide's toxicity [14, 15]. Furthermore, as mentioned in a preceding paragraph, cyanide is reportedly a carboxylase inhibitor [5]. Any of these agents, namely agents to which cyanide binds, may be suspected of acting as antigens when bound to cyanide. Having said this, also note that it may be possible to be immunologically sensitive to cyanide, and yet test negative for immunological sensitivity in laboratory testing, due to limitations in collecting various types of proteins to use in the preparation of antigenic solutions.

In light of the previous information, the fact that cyanide may bind to phosphatase is of key interest since autoantibodies in Type 1 Diabetes are directed against tyrosine phosphatases [13]. Of further interest is the fact that the A chain of the insulin molecule contains a disulfide bridge that may be vulnerable to reduction by cyanide. Breakage of the disulfide bridge on the A chain of insulin may negate the biological activity of insulin [11], causing what would seem to be insulin resistance since the insulin fails to function properly. Additionally, and of pertinence in regard to autoimmunity to insulin, the cyanide-bound insulin molecule may be antigenic.

Cyanide is present to at least some degree in all of the troposphere, with levels in industrialized regions expectedly higher [16]. There is marked variability in cyanide metabolism between individuals, so it is reasonable to conclude that tissue levels of cyanide will vary markedly between individuals, even when exposure to atmospheric cyanide for those individuals is the same.

Of note, 20% of patients with Type 1 Diabetes also have Autoimmune Thyroiditis [17]. With autoimmune thyroiditis, antibodies are directed against microsomal thyroid peroxidase, thyroglobulin, and the thyroid receptor for thyroid-stimulating hormone (TSH) [18]. As pointed out previously, cyanide reportedly binds to peroxidase [14]. Furthermore, thyroglobulin may have one or more disulfide bridges, somewhat comparable to the disulfide bridge on the A chain of insulin, and such disulfide bridges may be vulnerable to reduction by cyanide, especially considering that thyroglobulin contains approximately 240 half-cystine residues, almost all forming disulfide bonds [19]. Notably, a propensity for cyanide to act as a hapten may sometimes be increased due to genetic differences between individuals, and this may explain why so many persons with type 1 diabetes also have autoimmune thyroidities.

In speaking directly with a research representative of the American Diabetes Association, the author learned that diabetes has existed since ancient times, and that diabetes occurs in rural as well as urban areas. So far as diabetes from cyanide pollution is concerned, the author considers it pertinent that diabetes is seen more often in populations who move from rural to urban settings, and that the prevalence of diabetes appears to have increased over the past 50 years [20]. Major sources of cyanide pollution, such as vehicular exhaust and industry, are typically concentrated more in urban areas; and therefore, one would expect more diabetes in urban areas if cyanide is the cause. The author also considers it pertinent that diabetes occurs more often in women and in lower socioeconomic groups [20]. In dealing with populations of persons exhibiting overt symptoms of cyanide intoxication, the author has observed that, on the average, women seem to be somewhat more vulnerable to illness from cyanide pollution than men—perhaps due to smaller livers and/or enzyme differences (*though men are certainly affected, sometimes extremely*). Also, persons of lower socioeconomic status may be more likely to live in higher pollution areas; more likely to be exposed to higher concentrations of firsthand or secondhand cigarette smoke (*there are notably high concentrations of cyanide in cigarette smoke*); and more likely to have lower protein intake in their diets. Protein is mentioned because amino acids such as methionine, cysteine, and cystine play significant roles in the detoxification of cyanide; and nutritional deficiencies of protein (and also of vitamin B12) are associated with increased vulnerability to cyanide [21, 22, 23, 24].

The antiquity and rural existence of diabetes does not rule out cyanide as a causative factor. Cyanide may be released into the atmosphere from the burning of organic or synthetic compounds containing carbon and nitrogen, such as with the burning of fossil fuels. Thus, when mankind began using fire for cooking and heating, this accomplished the advent of air pollution containing cyanide—an advent that was compounded by the invention of smoking. Furthermore, over 2,650 plant species can produce hydrogen cyanide when eaten, including edible plants such as almonds, pits from stone fruits, sorghum, cassava, soybeans, spinach, lima beans, sweet potatoes, maize, millet, sugarcane, and bamboo shoots [25, 26, 27]. In the case of cassava, incomplete processing before consumption can actually result in acute cyanide toxicity; and as mentioned previously, dietary intake of cassava has been associated with an increased incidence of diabetes [4, 23]. Additionally, a genetic tendency toward diabetes is not in conflict with cyanide as a causative factor, since sensitivity to cyanide may sometimes be genetic. One genetic factor that would increase sensitivity to cyanide is when an individual inherits a deficiency of enzymes that are active in cyanide detoxification [22].

In 1997, it came to the author's attention that studies reveal an increased rate of non-insulin dependent diabetes among smokers [28, 29]. This is supportive of cyanide as the primary etiology of diabetes since there is an appreciable quantity of cyanide in cigarette smoke [30]. The risk of diabetes increases with the number of cigarettes smoked, and there appears to be an independent association between current smoking and insulin resistance [28, 29].

Insulin resistance decreases with the cessation of smoking, but it does not decrease to the level of persons who have never smoked [28]. This finding supports the hypothesis that higher exposures to cyanide in persons who become sensitive or vulnerable to cyanide may increase the deleterious effects that those persons experience from lower exposures to cyanide in the future (*as from air pollution*). There is published literature indicating that previously unaffected persons may develop vulnerability to illness from cyanide exposure, and that those persons will then continue to experience illness from repeated exposures to cyanide thereafter [31]. Mechanisms by which cyanide may induce insulin resistance include reduction of the disulfide bridge of the A chain of the insulin molecule, and may also include the binding of cyanide to tyrosine kinase.

Another interesting statistical finding was that men who consumed about two to four alcoholic drinks per day had a decreased rate of non-insulin dependent diabetes [28]. It was noted that insulin sensitivity (*insulin sensitivity is a good thing; whereas, insulin resistance is a bad thing*) was increased in persons who consumed one to three alcohol-containing drinks per day [28]. This is of notable interest since alcoholic beverages may contain several components that bind cyanide or function in the metabolism of cyanide. Two of the components that may be present in alcoholic beverages and that may bind cyanide are pyruvic acid (or pyruvate) and alpha-ketoglutaric acid (or alpha-ketoglutarate) [32, 33]. Two other components that may be present in alcoholic beverages and that may also bind cyanide are oxaloacetic acid (or oxaloacetate) and pyridoxal 5'-phosphate (vitamin B6) [33]. Another interesting fact is that drinking four or more cups of coffee a day reduces chances of diabetes, and the author hypothesizes that acids found in coffee may bind cyanide.

Thus, the fact that alcoholic beverages are protective against diabetes is supportive of cyanide as the etiology of diabetes. Furthermore, such findings suggest that treatment of the underlying cause of diabetes may reduce or prevent the occurrence of diabetes.

In speaking with a nurse at the International Diabetes Center of Tennessee, the author learned that persons with the inherited tendency to develop adult-onset diabetes also have the inherited tendency to become obese. Furthermore, this nurse stated that increased fatty weight causes increased insulin resistance in persons who develop adult-onset diabetes. This data is consistent with the hypothesis that cyanide is the underlying etiology of diabetes.

Cyanide may cause decreased metabolism of adipose tissue into glycerol for gluconeogenesis since glycerokinase (*glycerokinase is required in the metabolism of adipose tissue to form glycerol for gluconeogenesis*) requires ATP, and cyanide is noted to decrease the concentration of ATP [6, 7]. This may explain an increased propensity toward obesity in persons who metabolize cyanide poorly, though the author has also noted significant weight loss when cyanide sensitivity is severe. Additionally, cyanide inhibits reactions in which pyridoxal phosphate functions as a coenzyme; and deficiency of pyridoxal phosphate—which may be expected to yield similar results to inhibition of pyridoxal phosphate—results in a decrease in the neurotransmitters serotonin and GABA [6, 34, 35]. Notably, researchers have identified serotonin as the key chemical involved in overeating: low serotonin levels reportedly drive people to eat excessively [36]. Thus, given that poor metabolism of cyanide may be inherited, and that cyanide may induce both obesity and adult-onset diabetes, the inherited tendency for both obesity and adult-onset diabetes may result from inherited deficiencies in cyanide metabolism. This does not count out the possibility that obesity and diabetes may result from environmentally induced deficiencies of cyanide metabolism in persons who have no family history of diabetes.

Reportedly, a 10% weight loss is enough to see a reduction in the risk of diabetes; and as mentioned in a preceding paragraph, increased fatty weight is an apparent cause of increased insulin resistance [36]. During respiration at rest, added weight in the form of fat results in a higher level of alveolar ventilation in order to maintain the same arterial gas tensions that would be maintained at a lower level of alveolar ventilation if the same person were less fat [37]. A major source of cyanide is the inhalation of polluted air (*in the author's opinion, airborne cyanide is by far the most significant source of cyanide exposure*), so persons with increased alveolar ventilation would have increased delivery of cyanide to their bloodstream and tissues via the lungs [2]. Mechanisms by which cyanide may cause insulin resistance have been previously addressed, so increased delivery of cyanide to tissues secondary to obesity may explain the phenomenon of increased insulin resistance with increased fatty weight. Furthermore, the phenomenon of gestational diabetes may, at least in part, be explained by the fact that there is an increased minute volume during pregnancy (*minute volume is the amount of air inspired and expired in 1 minute*) [38]. Thus, women who metabolize cyanide poorly and who are thereby genetically inclined toward adult-onset diabetes may experience increased insulin resistance during pregnancy due to increased respiration and increased delivery of cyanide to body tissues. Such a hypothesis is consistent with the previously reported finding that the risk of diabetes increases with the number of cigarettes smoked, since increasing the number of cigarettes smoked increases the delivery of cyanide to the tissues [29]. And, although it is true that there is increased respiration for short periods of time during exercise, exercise results in the production of lactic acid which is converted to pyruvic acid [43], and pyruvic acid serves, to some degree, as an antidote for cyanide [46]. And furthermore, exercise contributes to the maintenance of proper weight, and probably contributes in other ways that reduce the effects of cyanide and reduce the incidence of diabetes [42].

Persons with diabetes suffer from peripheral neuropathy; and of note, chronic exposure to low doses of cyanide is associated with visual loss, ataxia, and other neurological problems [22, 33]. Also of note, in an animal study, hydroxocobalamin prevented demyelination in the central nervous system when given simultaneously with KCN (potassium cyanide) injections over a period of three weeks [22]. Persons with diabetes suffer kidney disease; and of note, in animal studies that focused upon effects of cyanide upon the kidney, proliferation of glomerular cells, an increase in absolute kidney weight, vacuolation, swelling, proximal tubule damage with desquamation of the epithelium, urinary casts, and increased urinary protein have all been noted [39, 40, 41].

Vitamin B6 (pyridoxal phosphate) serves as an example of an agent that is inhibited by the binding of cyanide; and by virtue of such binding, vitamin B6 is also useful in treating cyanide intoxication [6, 33]. It would seem logical, then, that if cyanide binds to the disulfide bridge on the A chain of insulin, thereby causing inhibition and insulin resistance; then aggressive, continuous treatment with insulin may also serve, to some degree, as a treatment for cyanide intoxication. This may explain, at least in part, why more aggressive, continuous control of hyperglycemia (*using insulin*) in diabetes seems to decrease the severity of the disease. However, treatment with agents such as sodium thiosulfate pentahydrate, alpha-ketoglutaric acid, and hydroxocobalamin may yield far better results than the use of insulin alone. Furthermore, the use of agents such as alpha-ketoglutaric acid, hydroxocobalamin, and sodium thiosulfate pentahydrate in the diets of children and adults with genetic risks for diabetes may greatly reduce the incidence of this disease.

A preceding paragraph addressed the fact that cyanide may inhibit enzymes by binding to metallic cofactors, such as chromium [8]. The fact that cyanide may bind to certain metals may enable those metals to serve in treating cyanide poisoning. Cobalt, although itself toxic in some forms, has been observed to act as a chelator in treating cyanide poisoning [22]. The author surmises that chromium, and also vanadium, likely serve to some degree as chelators in treating cyanide intoxication.

Additionally, it has been noted that increased dietary intake of any one of three other metals, namely potassium, calcium, or magnesium, decreased the incidence of adult-onset diabetes [44].

In pigs fed cassava (*one of the more significant foods that can produce cyanide inside the body when eaten*) for 110 days, a proliferation of glomerular cells in the kidney was noted upon histopathological examination [39]. This appears significant since the most striking and specific vascular changes found in diabetes take place in the smallest vessels, such as in the capillaries where thickening of the basement membranes occurs—and the most striking example of this thickening is in the glomerulus of the kidney [19]. Additionally, the major arteries of diabetic individuals are prone to atheromatous changes that are indistinguishable from such changes in nondiabetic individuals, except that these changes occur earlier and more extensively in diabetic individuals [19]. Such proneness toward atherosclerosis in diabetic individuals may result from poor cyanide metabolism and resultant decreased cystathionine synthase activity, with cyanide inhibiting pyridoxal phosphate which serves as the coenzyme (*a coenzyme is a nonprotein, organic compound that is necessary for the functioning of an enzyme*) for cystathionine synthase (*an enzyme*) [19, 6]. Reduced cystathionine synthase activity (*such as seen in hereditary deficiency or absence of this enzyme*) leads to a block in the catabolism (*breakdown*) of homocysteine [19]. Investigators at the Harvard School of Public Health report that elevated serum levels of homocysteine inhibit endothelial cell growth and have a pro-oxidant proliferative effect on smooth muscle cell growth—hallmarks of arteriosclerosis—by activating genes governing the cell cycle [45].

The binding of cyanide to vitamin B6 occurs because cyanide binds to the carbonyl group of pyridoxal phosphate [6, 33]. Of note, in what is referred to as *folding* in the formation of proteins, both the helix and the beta-sheet structures are held together by hydrogen–bonding interactions between the amide nitrogen on one amino acid and the carbonyl oxygen (*the oxygen atom of a carbonyl group*) on another amino acid [47]. The author hypothesizes that cyanide may bind to carbonyl groups during the process of protein folding; and thus, cause misfolding of protein (*protein folding is the physical process by which a protein chain is translated to its native three-dimensional structure, typically a "folded" conformation, by which the protein becomes biologically functional [48]*). And of interest, misfolding of protein is thought to be a factor in several diseases, including autism [49], Alzheimer's disease, Parkinson's disease, and diabetes [50]. And as might be expected, there is increased Alzheimer's disease in persons with diabetes [51], and increased Parkinson's disease in persons with diabetes [52]; and persons with autism are more likely to develop Type 2 Diabetes [53].

In summary, cyanide may play a key role in adult-onset diabetes due to toxic effects that are totally unrelated to autoimmunity. Additionally, cyanide may play a key role in Type 1 Diabetes where autoimmunity does exist. In both cases, regular treatment for environmental cyanide sensitivity may lower tissue cyanide levels and prove beneficial to health.

<u>References</u>:

1.) Prasenjit Manna, Joydeep Das, Parames C. Sil. *Role of Sulfur Containing Amino Acids as an Adjuvant Therapy in the Prevention of Diabetes and its Associated Complications*. Current Diabetes Reviews Volume 9, Issue 3, 2013.

2.) Oesch TR. Presentation at the 1995 International Congress on Hazardous Waste: Impact on Human and Ecological Health, Atlanta Georgia, Sponsored by U.S. Department of Health and Human Services, Public Health Service, Agency for Toxic Substances and Disease Registry.

3.) Anonymous. *Diabetes, cyanide, and rat poison* [editorial]. Lancet. 2(8138):341-2, 1979 Aug 18.

4.) Davidson JC. *Cyanide, cassava, and diabetes* [letter]. Lancet. 2(8143):635, 1979 Sep 22.

5.) De Metz M, Soute BAM, Hemker HC, Vermeer C. *The inhibition of Vitamin K-Dependent Carboxylase by Cyanide*. FEBS Lett 137(2):253-256, January 1982.

6.) Isom GE, Liu DHW, Way JL. *Effect of Sublethal Doses of Cyanide on Glucose Catabolism*. Biochem Pharmacol 24(8):871-5, 1975.

7.) Martin DW, Mayes PA, Rodwell VW, Granner DK. Harper's Review of Biochemistry, Twentieth Edition. Los Altos, California: Lange Medical Publications, 1985, pp. 107, 164, 185, & 187.

8.) Way JL. *Cyanide intoxication and its mechanism of antagonism.* Ann Rev Pharmacol Toxicol 24:451-481, 1984.

9.) Thorn GW, Adams RD, Braunwald E, Isselbacher KJ, Petersdorf RG. Harrison's Principles of Internal Medicine, Eighth Edition. New York, London, etc.: McGraw-Hill Book Company, 1977, p. 468.

10.) Kapil V, Keogh J. United States Department of Health & Human Services, Public Health Service, Agency for Toxic Substances and Disease Registry. Case Studies in Environmental Medicine, Chromium Toxicity, June 1990.

11.) Goth A. Medical Pharmacology, Sixth Edition. St. Louis: C. V. Mosby Company, 1972, pp. 438, & 440.

12.) Norris JC, Utley WS, Hume AS. *Mechanism of Antagonizing Cyanide-Induced Lethality by alpha-Ketoglutaric Acid.* Toxicology 62, 275-283, 1990.

13.) Norris JM, Beaty B, Klingensmith G, Yu L, Hoffman M, Chase HP, Erlich HA, Hamman RF, Eisenbarth GS, Rewers M. *Lack of Association Between Early Exposure to Cow's Milk Protein and B-Cell Autoimmunity.* JAMA, August 28, 1996—Vol. 276, No. 8, pp. 609-14.

14.) Ardelt BK, Borowitz JL, Isom GE. Brain lipid peroxidation and antioxidant protectant mechanisms following acute cyanide intoxication. Toxicology 56:147-154, 1989.

15.) Rieders F. *Noxious gases and vapors I: Carbon monoxide, cyanides, methemoglobin, and sulfhemoglobin.* In: DePalma JR, ed. Drill's pharmacology in medicine, 4th ed. New York, NY: McGraw-Hill Book Company, 1180-1205, 1971.

16.) Cicerone RJ, Zellner R. *The atmospheric chemistry of hydrogen cyanide* (HCN). J Geophy Res 88:10689-10696, 1983.

17.) Van Meter QL. Clinical Professor of Pediatrics, Emory University School of Medicine, Atlanta. Audio-Digest Foundation, Family Practice, Volume 44, Number 44, November 25, 1996.

18.) Robinson DR. *Immunologic Tolerance and Autoimmunity.* Scientific American, Medicine, Volume 2, 6:VI:8.

19.) Bondy PK, Rosenberg LE. *METABOLIC CONTROL AND DISEASE*, Eighth Edition. Philadelphia/London/Toronto: W. B. Saunders Company, 1980, pp. 319, 662-3, & 1329.

20.) Diabetes statistics. In: Cowie CC, Eberhardt MS, eds. American Diabetes Association's Diabetes 1996: Vital Statistics. Alexandria, Va: American Diabetes Association; 1996:13-20.

21.) Wilson, J. *Leber's hereditary optic atrophy: A possible defect of cyanide metabolism.* Clin Sci 29:505-515, 1983.

22.) Baumeister RGH, Schievelbien H, Zickgraf-Rudel G. *Toxicological and Clinical Aspects of Cyanide Metabolism.* Arzneim-Forsch. (Drug Res.) 25, Nr. 7 (1975), pp. 1056-1063.

23.) Mlingi N, Poulter NH, Rosling H. *An outbreak of acute intoxications from consumption of insufficiently processed cassava in Tanzania.* NUTR RES 12(6):677-687, 1992.

24.) Tylleskar T, Banea M, Bikangi N, et al. *Cassava cyanogens and konzo, an upper motoneuron disease found in Africa* [published erratum appears in Lancet 1992 Feb 15;339(8790):440]. Lancet 339(8787):208-211, 1992.

25.) Seigler DS. *Cyanide and cyanogenic glycosides.* In: G.A. Rosenthal, M.R. Berenbaum, eds. Herbivores: their interaction with secondary plant metabolites. Academic Press, New York, N.Y. 35-77, 1991.

26.) Swain E, LI CP, Poulton JE. *Development of the potential for cyanogenesis in maturing black cherry* (Prunus serotina Ehrh.) fruits. Plant Physiol (Bethesda) 98(4):1423-1428, 1992.

27.) Fiksel J, Cooper C, Eschenroeder A, et al. *Exposure and risk assessment for cyanide.* EPA/440/4-85/008. NTIS PB85-220572, 1981.

28.) Rimm EB, Chan J, Stampfer MJ, Colditz GA, Willett. *Prospective study of cigarette smoking, alcohol use, and the risk of diabetes in men.* BMJ 1995;310:555-9.

29.) Rimm EB, Manson JE, Stampfer MJ, Colditz GA, Willett WC, Rosner B, Hennekens CH, Speizer FE. *Cigarette Smoking and the Risk of Diabetes in Women.* American Journal of Public Health, February 1993, Vol. 83, No. 2.

30.) Djuric D, Raicevic P, Konstantinovic I. *Excretion of Thiocyanates in Urine of Smokers*. Archives of Environmental Health, Vol. 5, July '62, pp. 20-21.

31.) Hamilton A, Hardy HL. Cyanides. Industrial Toxicology, 3rd Edition. Acton, Massachusetts: Publishing Sciences Group, Inc., 1974, pp. 224-7.

32.) Amerine MA, Berg HW, Cruess WV. *The Technology of Wine Making*, third edition. Westport, Connecticut: The Avi Publishing Company, Inc., 1972, pp. 189-90, & 211.

33.) U.S. Department of Health & Human Services, Public Health Service, Agency for Toxic Substances and Disease Registry. *Toxicological Profile for Cyanide*, TP-92/09, April 1993, p. 57. (Prepared by: Syracuse Research Corporation Under Subcontract to: Clement International Corporation Under Contract No. 205-88-0608.)

34.) Dakshinamurti K, LeBlancq WD, Herchi R, Haulicek V. *Brain monoamines of pyridoxine-deficient growing rats*. Exp. Brain Res. 26:355-66, 1976.

35.) Dakshinamurti K, Paulose CS, Siow YL. *Neurobiology of pyridoxine*. In: Reynolds RD, Leklem JE. Vitamin B-6: Its Role in Health and Disease. New York: Alan R. Liss, Inc., pp. 99-121, 1985.

36.) Shelton DL. *Pharmacological fat-fighters*. American Medical News/March 3, 1997, p. 13.

37.) Bates DV, Christie RV. *Respiratory Function in Disease*. Philadelphia & London: W. B. Saunders Company, 1965, p. 104.

38.) Niswander KR. *Obstetrics, Essentials of Clinical Practice*, first edition. Boston: Little, Brown and Company, 1976, p. 46.

39.) Tewe OO, Maner JH. *Performance and pathophysiological changes in pregnant pigs fed cassava diets containing different levels of cyanide*. Res Vet Sci 30:147-151, 1981b.

40.) NTP. National Toxicology Program *Technical Report on toxicity studies of sodium cyanide* (CAS No. 143-33-9) administered in drinking water to F344/N rats and B6C3F1 mice, NIH Publication 94-3386. U.S. Department of Health and Human Services, Public Health Service, National Institutes of Health., 1993.

41.) Kamalu BP. *Pathological changes in growing dogs fed on a balanced cassava* (Manihot esculenta Crantz) diet. BR J Nutr 69(3):921-934, 1992.

42.) Manson JE, Rimm EB, Stampfer MJ, Colditz GA, Willett WC, Krolewski AS, Rosner B, Hennekens CH, Speizer FE. *Physical activity and incidence of non-insulin-dependent diabetes mellitus in women*. Lancet 1991; 338:774-78.

43.) Guyton AC. *BASIC HUMAN PHYSIOLOGY: NORMAL FUNCTION AND MECHANISMS OF DISEASE*, first edition. Philadelphia-London-Toronto: W. B. Saunders Company, 1971, pp. 563, & 581.

44.) Colditz GA, Manson JE, Stampfer MJ, Rosner B, Willett WC, Speizer FE. *Diet and risk of clinical diabetes in women*. Am J Nutr 1992;55:1018-23.

45.) Lee AM. *Lipoprotein Patterns, Plaque, Homocysteine, and Hormones Among Ongoing Cardiology Studies. Pro-oxidant Homocysteine*. JAMA, October 9, 1996—Vol. 276, No. 14, p. 1124.

46.) *Cyanide inhibition and pyruvate-induced recovery of cytochrome c oxidase*, Hana Nůsková [1], Marek Vrbacký, Zdeněk Drahota, Josef Houštěk, J Bioenerg Biomembr 2010 Oct;42(5):395-403. doi: 10.1007/s10863-010-9307-6. Epub 2010 Aug 20.

47.) *Levels of Protein Structure*. (2020, May 30). Retrieved August 28, 2021, from https://chem.libretexts.org/@go/page/46046

48.) Alberts B, Johnson A, Lewis J, Raff M, Roberts K, Walters P (2002). *"The Shape and Structure of Proteins"*. *Molecular Biology of the Cell;* Fourth Edition. New York and London: Garland Science. ISBN 978-0-8153-3218-3.

49.) De Jaco A, Lin MZ, Dubi N, et al. *Neuroligin trafficking deficiencies arising from mutations in the alpha/beta-hydrolase fold protein family. J Biol Chem*. 2010;285(37):28674-28682. doi:10.1074/jbc.M110.139519

50.) Mukherjee A, Morales-Scheihing D, Butler PC, Soto C. *Type 2 diabetes as a protein misfolding disease*. Trends Mol Med. 2015 Jul;21(7):439-49. doi: 10.1016/j.molmed.2015.04.005. Epub 2015 May 18. PMID: 25998900; PMCID: PMC4492843.

51.) Biessels GJ, Kappelle LJ; Utrecht Diabetic Encephalopathy Study Group. *Increased risk of Alzheimer's disease in Type II diabetes: insulin resistance of the brain or insulin-induced amyloid pathology?* Biochem Soc Trans. 2005 Nov;33(Pt 5):1041-4. doi: 10.1042/BST0331041. PMID: 16246041.

52.) Cheong JLY, de Pablo-Fernandez E, Foltynie T, Noyce AJ. *The Association Between Type 2 Diabetes Mellitus and Parkinson's Disease. J Parkinsons Dis.* 2020;10(3):775-789. doi:10.3233/JPD-191900

53.) Chen MH, Lan WH, Hsu JW, Huang KL, Su TP, Li CT, Lin WC, Tsai CF, Tsai SJ, Lee YC, Chen YS, Pan TL, Chang WH, Chen TJ, Bai YM. *Risk of Developing Type 2 Diabetes in Adolescents and Young Adults With Autism Spectrum Disorder: A Nationwide Longitudinal Study.* Diabetes Care. 2016 May;39(5):788-93. doi: 10.2337/dc15-1807. Epub 2016 Mar 22. PMID: 27006513.

* * * * * * *

In closing, the author considers the best test for chronic illness caused by environmental cyanide intoxication to be a trial of treatment; and therefore, he considers the first chapter of this book to be very important. Persons who desire more information in regard to airborne cyanide and its effects upon human health may refer to a much larger book entitled, *A Breath of Cyanide*, by Timothy Swiss.